CONNIE WILLIAMS

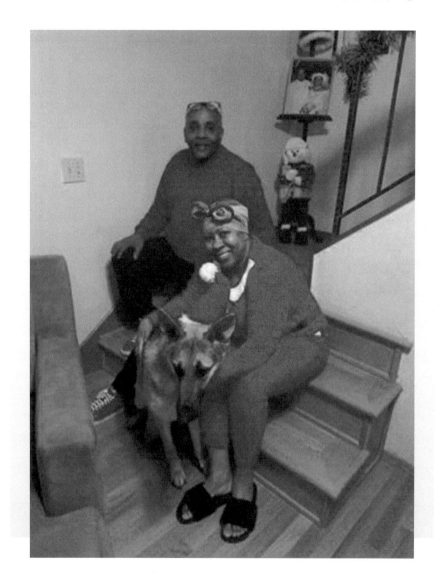

In Sickness and In Health

In Sickness and In Health

iUniverse books may be ordered through booksellers or by contacting:

iUniverse
1663 Liberty Drive
Bloomington, IN 47403
www.iuniverse.com
844-349-9409

Because of the dynamic nature of the Internet, any web addresses or links contained in this book may have changed since publication and may no longer be valid. The views expressed in this work are solely those of the author and do not necessarily reflect the views of the publisher, and the publisher hereby disclaims any responsibility for them.

Any people depicted in stock imagery provided by Getty Images are models, and such images are being used for illustrative purposes only. Certain stock imagery © Getty Images.

Scripture quotations marked KJV are from the Holy Bible, King James Version (Authorized Version). First published in 1611. Quoted from the KJV Classic Reference Bible, Copyright © 1983 by The Zondervan Corporation.

ISBN: 978-1-6632-3056-0 (sc)
978-1-6632-3057-7 (e)

Library of Congress Control Number: 2021921400

Print information available on the last page.

iUniverse rev. date: 11/15/2021

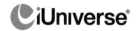

In Sickness and In Health

Acknowledgements

We are grateful to the ER team at St. Joseph's Hospital, including Dr. H, and Nurses: Terri, Dionne, Patsy, Mary Lou, and Kirby. Their ability to assess, administer, and care for my husband in such a critical moment was exceptional, and is highly appreciative. Our Special thanks to: Mariam, Lief, Scott, Crista, Bonnie, Ilhann, Alicia, Michelle, Julie, Kara, Lacee, May, Steph, Uche, and Katie, for their awesome caregiving during his hospitalization.

Many thanks to the care team of office staff, nurses, and therapists at Fairview Acute Rehabilitation Center: Ousman, Dan, Matt, Maura, Katelyn, and Sharon, for the extraordinary care they provided. At the start of each shift, they would come into the room, introduce themselves, check Tony's vitals, and would ask if we needed anything. They were extremely attentive to our needs.

Much gratitude to the team of doctors who played such a crucial role in Tony's health care and continues to evaluate him to this day: Dr. H. Aggarwal, Neurologist, Dr. G. Knudsen, MD, and Dr. P. Salehi, MD, Physical Medicine and Rehabilitation.

To our dear family, friends, and business associates, thank you for your outpouring of love and support through your prayers, phone calls, cards, text messages, and visits during this difficult time.

Appreciation to Freddie Thomas for his contributions to this manuscript's edits and release.

Finally, to the most amazing husband of 27 wonderful years! Together with God, we have been through life's challenges and storms and were able to overcome and now walk in victory. I thank God for giving you the strength and will power to work hard on your recovery. You continued to push through even on those days when it was tough, maintaining a positive mindset and always giving thanks to God. Twenty-seven years ago, we promised God and each other in marriage to love and respect, honor and cherish, and to care for each other in sickness and health, and in prosperity and adversity, for as long as we both shall live. I am blessed and proud to call you my friend, my lover, my husband. Today we make this same declaration as a testimony, giving God all the glory and thanking Him for our next assignment.

Table of Contents

Introduction

On Tuesday morning, July 16, 2019, we thought we were going to St. Joseph's Hospital Emergency Room for a minor ailment, but it turned out to be a life-changing event. At age 57, my husband had suffered a severe stroke. Our lives as we knew them were shattered, and a new chapter began.

The next eight days in the hospital, confined to a private room and in perpetual prayer, seemed like eight weeks. I stayed near my husband the entire time. Most of my time was spent observing every action taken by doctors, neurologist, nurses, therapists, and other clinicians. I asked many questions to broaden my knowledge and understanding of what a stroke patient goes through, and I kept a diary, noting every time the nurse entered the room to check his vitals, draw blood, administer medications, etc.

Anyone who has ever spent time in the hospital knows that it is not a relaxing experience. Every 30 minutes, a nurse will enter the room to check the patient's vitals and perform any other tests ordered by the doctor. When you have finally fallen asleep and are resting, you hear the door open and awaken to see the light from the hallway. Of course, because I stayed in the room with my husband, I was awakened as well.

I share this story and important information to raise awareness, educate, and equip the readers with some fundamental knowledge and understanding of the silent, yet fatal disease of stroke before it catches you off guard and interrupts your life. Perhaps you know someone close to you who has been impacted by such a life-altering disruption of a stroke; you do not have to follow the same path. Make the choice to change your lifestyle and eating habits to live a healthier life.

Chapter 1

Recognizing the Signs

The American Stroke Association defines stroke as a disease that affects the arteries leading to and within the brain. It occurs when blood clots form in the artery and blocks the normal blood circulation to any part of the brain, preventing the brain tissue from receiving enough blood, oxygen, and nutrients. If blood flow to a part of the brain is interrupted, the brain can suffer permanent damage within a short time, resulting in disability or even death. Therefore, when someone has a stroke, time is vital. The sooner you get to the hospital; the faster doctors can administer emergency medical treatment, the less damage there will be to the brain tissue, and the better your chances of recovery. Your survival and recovery will depend on how quickly you get medical attention, the type of stroke, and the area of the brain affected.

Early detection of stroke symptoms is critical. Some of the most common symptoms are: difficulty speaking, sudden numbness or weakness of the arm, leg, or face, particularly on one side of the body, sudden blurred or decreased vision in one or both eyes, trouble speaking, understanding speech or reading, loss of physical balance or coordination, dizziness, severe headache, fainting or seizures. Some of these warning signs may last for only a brief period then disappear and reappear. If you notice someone exhibit any of these symptoms, immediately call 911 or take them to the nearest hospital emergency room, whichever is faster!

Stroke, according to the American Stroke Association, is the fifth leading cause of death and a leading cause of disability in the United States. African Americans, are two to three times more likely than Whites to have a stroke, more likely to suffer a stroke at a younger age, have a higher mortality rate, and often take longer to recover than Whites, says the National Institute of Neurological Disorders and Stroke (NINDS). Further research claims that African American women have the highest stroke rates of all! Yes, you heard clearly!

How do we combat this illness? We must make lifestyle changes immediately—diet and exercise! Check in with your doctor on a regular basis for physical exams and monitor your blood pressure and cholesterol levels. Because red meat is high in cholesterol, fat, and sodium content, all of which are established risk factors that cause blockages in blood vessels, which can lead to heart disease and stroke, you should restrict red meat intake in your diet. Carbohydrate-rich foods should be consumed in moderation. Look for products that are made from whole grains, and make vegetables the main part of the meal.

Regular exercise routine is also key. The American Heart Association recommends that adults get at least 150 minutes of moderately intense or at least 75 minutes of vigorous physical exercise each week. Walk at the least 30-minutes a day. Making these small changes will add great improvements on your health and quality of life. If you want to live, you must make this lifestyle change!

Chapter 2

A Life-Changing Moment

July 16, 2019 began a new chapter in our lives. We arrived home for the evening after a night of celebration for my sister-in-law receiving the prestigious Lewis Sports Foundation award. I began to close blinds as my husband proceeded upstairs. About midway up the stairs, he tripped. The sound was so loud that I inquired if he was okay. He replied yes, he was tired and going to bed.

As we slept through the night, Tony awaken around 2:00 a.m., got up and went to the bathroom. At that time, he said his leg felt different. Around 5:00 a.m., he awoke again and went to the bathroom. As he was getting back onto bed, I awoke, and he said to me that he did not like the way his leg felt; he said it felt heavy and he was almost dragging it. He asked me to login on the iPad to check the status of one of our restaurants. After completing the process, he then told me he needed to go to the hospital emergency room. As we prepared to get up and dress, I went down stairs to allow Leah, our two-year old German Shepard, out, while Tony work his way down stairs on his own. I assisted him out of the house by having him hold onto my shoulder while we walked off the deck and into the garage on our way to the ER.

Upon arrival to the ER, Tony walked up to the front desk, answered the receptionist's questions then took a seat to complete an intake form. As he gripped the pen to begin writing, we realized he was not able to write. The nurse quickly turned around and spoke to two individuals standing behind her. They sprung into swift action, with one of them grabbing a wheelchair and meeting us on the front side of the desk. They rushed Tony to the back where doctors and nurses immediately began urgent care by getting him in bed, undressing and putting on a gown, connecting him to monitors, and performing medical evaluations. Tony was able to follow all of the doctor's commands during the exams. His blood pressure was elevated, so they began giving him medication to lower it. After a while, the doctor returned for further evaluations and instructed him to follow more commands, which he was able to do all of the commands as requested. A few hours later, Tony looked up to see the words "admitted stroke" written on the whiteboard directly above my head where I sat. I quickly turned and looked up at the board and read the same thing! The nurses and doctors that came in and out of the room, however, never mentioned a stroke, which I'm sure was done by design to not alarm the patient.

Throughout this process, I remained calm, making spiritual declarations, and praying silently for God's intervention. The first person I called was my sister-in-law, Deborah (Deb). The reason I called her first is that in life, you must always have a person who is in Christ, strong in their faith, knows how to call on the name of Jesus, and a prayer warrior. You don't need anyone who will panic and runoff with incorrect, incomplete information, speaking negative words that give power to the work of the enemy. A person with that mindset thinks only about other people who have gone through similar difficulties in their lives and talks about how it damaged their physical and emotional well-being, and how bad they are, and how they have become disabled. They don't recall those who suffered this type of interruption and overcame against all odds. Therefore, in every case, we've learned the most important lesson, in every situation, is Don't Panic! This is the foundation of our spiritual education!

Following an overnight stay at the hospital when the doctor visited, Tony was no longer able to respond to his directives. It was evident then that he'd had a stroke on the left side of his brain. The injury effected his capacity to move the right side of his body and caused some speech difficulty. Thank God, he had no memory loss or other adverse effects, which can happen when the stroke occurs on the left side of the brain.

Chapter 3

Types of Strokes

The American Heart Association classifies strokes into four categories: Ischemic Stroke, Transient Ischemic Attack, Hemorrhagic Stroke, and Cryptogenic Stroke. Ischemic Stroke happens when blood flow to a part of the brain is blocked. The blood clot could form in one of the brain's arteries or elsewhere in the body and then travel to the brain. It accounts for approximately 80% of all strokes.

Transient Ischemic Attack (TIA) is called a mini stroke. The symptoms are the same as for a stroke, but they tend to go away in less than an hour. A TIA leaves no lasting effect on the brain, but it serves as a warning that you are at risk for a major stroke at any time. Even if your symptoms have subsided or disappeared, you should seek medical attention right away.

Hemorrhagic Stroke is when a weaken blood vessel in or near the brain ruptures, causing bleeding into the brain. Pressure from the blood injures the brain cells, and the burst vessel no longer supplies blood to the area of the brain it serves. The most common cause is uncontrolled high blood pressure. Trauma can also cause Hemorrhagic Stroke.

A clot that restricts the blood from flowing to the brain is the most common cause of a stroke. However, it is not always possible to pinpoint the cause of the stroke. The American Heart Association termed this type a Cryptogenic Stroke. Some studies suggest that African Americans and Hispanics have a higher risk of Cryptogenic Stroke.

Regardless of the types of strokes, there are preventable health measures you can take to control and reduce your risk. Here are a few:

- Develop a doctor/patient relationship with your healthcare provider and get regular check-ups

- Manage your blood pressure and cholesterol levels regularly

- Make physical activity and exercise a part of your daily routine

- Follow your doctor's instructions regarding medications

- Maintain a balanced diet, including low fat/low salt foods

- If you smoke, quit; if you don't, don't start

If you experience symptoms of a stroke or witness someone showing signs, You must act FAST!!! Remember the word, fast.

**F: Face – smile

Does one side of the face droop?

**A: ARMS - raise both arms

Does one drift downward?

**S: Speech - repeat a simple sentence

Are the words slurred?

Can he/ she repeat the sentence correctly?

**T: TIME - call 911 or get to the hospital fast

Brain cells are dying

Tony's interruption was caused by an ischemic stroke. Throughout his stay in the hospital from July 16-23, 2019, I would not leave his side. Each day I would go home for a shower, change of clothes and back at his side, encouraging and reminding him who he is in Christ, and God is able to do exceedingly, abundantly, above all we could ask are think according to the power that works within us. (Ephesians 3:20, King James Version)

Chapter 4

Journey to Recovery

Tony began physical therapy, occupational therapy, and speech therapy during his stay at St. Joseph's hospital. The doctors and nurses were amazed at his willpower and determination to work hard with his therapists after such drastic life-altering unexpected event that disrupted our plans for the next day and going forward.

Sometimes life throws us some curve balls that we aren't prepared for or understand, but with determination and the Word of God as the foundation to stand on, you do what you must, and it is what propels you to succeed. It may be a little hard in the beginning, but if you are in Christ, you make continuous declarations unto Him of His promises to those who walk upright and are faithful and continuously remind Him that His Word shall not return void. These and more comforting Words of God helped to strengthen us through this trial.

After nine days in St. Joseph's hospital, Tony's condition continued to improve, and he was given instructions to be discharged the following day. We were so excited! I began to pack up many of his belongings so the morning would go quickly before leaving.

The next morning the regular routine occurred with the nurse taking his vitals, breakfast, and doctor visit. Everything went well. The nurse came into the room at midday and went over the discharge papers. After signing, she gave us instructions and directions to be immediately discharged to Fairview Acute Rehabilitation Center.

As Tony prepared to get ready, with my assistance, he sat at the edge of the bed. When I asked him what was wrong, he stated he did not feel well. I requested a nurse to come and recheck his vitals, and she notified the doctor, who also returned. The doctor ordered blood work and other tests, and advised that Tony remain in the hospital another day for evaluation. While he was being taken for another MRI and other tests, I began to unpack my bags, and the nurse returned to the room with new admittance paperwork for me to complete. Thank God, all of the test results were negative.

The next morning we repeated the same procedure of filling out the discharge paperwork for immediate admission to Fairview Acute Rehabilitation Center. The instructions were firm and strict to go straight to the facility, where Tony's room was ready and the staff was waiting for him.

After being away from home for nine days, Tony missed seeing Leah. Once we were in the car our thought was to hop on the express, swing by the house, pull on the backside of the garage door, and I would run into the house and retrieve Leah so that she would know that Tony was okay. Leah sensed something wasn't quite right; Tony had been missing from home, and I was in and out of the house quickly each day, with very little time to cuddle, play ball, and chase her around the yard. But we were obedient to the strict doctors' order to go directly to the rehab center. Prior to reaching the destination, my phone rang, and it was the front desk at the rehab center, wanting to know our location. We were approaching the parking ramp, and I informed them we would be in shortly.

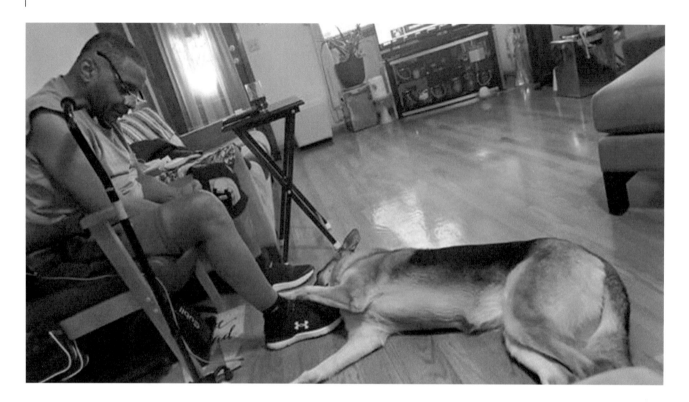

On our first day of therapy, we went through orientation. We were given a welcome handbook and literature on stroke patients to read at our leisure before being given a tour of the facility. We had a private room with a chair that converted into a twin size bed, allowing me to stay with him. The nurse provided me with the necessary bedding for a good night's sleep. As we were settling in, the nurse came in, took Tony's vitals, gave him his medications, and explained that someone else would be in to give us a schedule for occupational, physical, speech, and cognitive therapy, which would begin the next day.

We are now adjusting to life after the stroke. Tony's daily schedule was written on the whiteboard, beginning early morning at 7:00 a.m. with physical therapy, then a one-hour break before speech and cognitive therapy. It was followed by occupational therapy, another break, and occasionally a nap before another round of physical therapy for the day. This was our new routine for the next 16 days of Tony's stay.

During the first few days, the nurses came into the room on a regular basis to take his vitals. Sometimes just as I would close my eyes, I would hear the nurse enter the room to check his vitals or administer medications. Because Tony still required assistance getting out of bed and walking, only the nurse could assist him. They placed the alarm on his bed for him to buss them when he needed.

After much physical and occupational therapy, Tony was stronger and able to be challenged more during his sessions. Now, when he is in his room, he wants to be self-sufficient, despite the fact that he knows he should not get out of bed without the nurse's assistance.

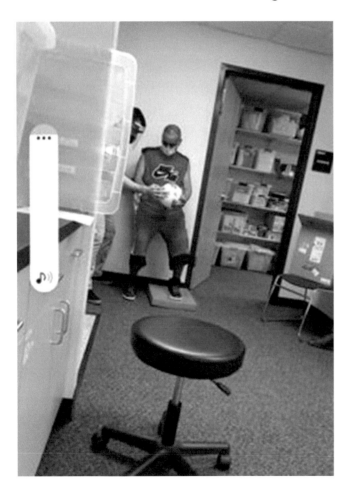

Tony would spend the next five days alone. It was the 2019 WNBA All-Star Game in Las Vegas, and my sister-in-law, niece, and I had reservations. Naturally, after this interruption, I tried to find someone else to bless with my reservation and ticket so that I could stay by my husband's side. After spending ten days at his side, he said to me, "I know you're trying to see how you can get out of going on your trip, you need to go. I will be okay, I want you to go and enjoy yourself." I went home and packed my carry-on bag. The next day I was off to Las Vegas.

Of course, we talked every day, many times a day. On the second day away from my husband, when I spoke with him, he told me he slid off the bed that morning while trying to put on his socks. His arms were not yet strong enough for him to get up on his own. Just as he fell, the nurse entered the room and radioed for help, "I got a fall, I got a fall." Two more nurses rushed in and helped him back onto the bed. He explained to them that he did not fall; instead, he was sitting at the edge of the bed attempting to put on his socks, when he slipped off due to the fabric of his shorts. The nurse checked him for bruises and again instructed him to use the bedside alarm to alert them when he needed to get up, which he did not like but understood the protocol was for his safety. I was ready to get on the next flight out as Tony was telling me this, but he convinced me the incident happened as he described and that he was fine.

Tony has now begun to wheel himself down to the shower, remove his clothes, move to the shower chair and wash himself. Being immobile on his right side and having to rely on his left hand was awkward at first, but he made progress every day. Everyday routine tasks that were second nature have become a challenge since the stroke. As he relearned to perform tasks on his own, the therapist would have to check off that he passed each test when he accomplished them, such as brushing his teeth, dressing himself, bathing himself, pronouncing words clearly, memory challenges, and so on.

I looked forward to the morning visits. I would arise; the nurse would come in, take Tony's vitals, and offer me a cup of coffee. As he doze off asleep again, I would pray and meditate while glancing out of the third floor window looking for the turkeys that would stroll about in the mornings with their young trailing behind, scratching and pecking for their breakfast.

Tony was evaluated after about four sessions of speech and cognitive therapy, and proven to have made sufficient progress, allowing him to be discharged. The time had finally arrived! Friday, August 16, 2019, my husband was released to come home! Before his discharge, we had to go through a checklist to ensure his safety once we were home. The checklist consisted of the proximity of the bathroom, access to the shower, his sleeping quarters, removal of any rugs and other items that might cause him to stumble or fall. Once at home we made immediate transitions for safety precautions. We added handrails into the main level bathroom, installed a higher toilet, put things at reach for easy access, etc.

As we transition to living on the main floor, I set up an automatic air mattress on legs, which would allow Tony to easily move around and get in and out of the bed. I placed the bed into the living room and slept on the couch next to him in case he needed anything. Because Tony's legs were weak and he had just begun walking, we did not want to risk him stumbling or falling in the middle of the night while going to or from the restroom. I was also hypersensitive to his every move, so whenever his made one, I jumped up and asked what was wrong. Even when he had to urinate, I would assist him in holding the urine bottle. If you do not consider yourself a humble person, this practice will undoubtable humble you if you have love in your heart for anyone. I continued this routine for a year.

After Tony's stay at the Minnesota Acute Rehabilitation Center, one of his main goals was to regain enough strength in his legs to walk our daughter down the aisle for her upcoming wedding. To do so, he worked hard at his physical and occupational outpatient therapy sessions, which he attended three to four days per week, as well as at home. In addition, I purchased him a Cubii Elliptical machine so he could ride it daily and set step goals and levels, which he constantly exceeded. At times, he would complain about how hard it was to get started, and I would encourage him that he could do it, and cycled alongside him. He always outpaced me! As he persevered through the therapy and grew stronger and stronger, the day came when he was able to walk our daughter down the aisle for her wedding, with the assistance of a quad cane.

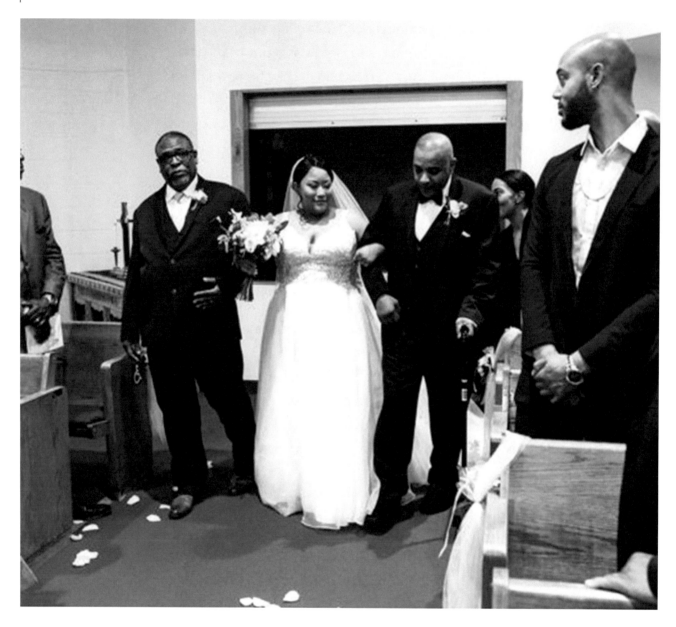

Tony continues his outpatient physical therapy, pool therapy, and riding the FES bike, while focusing on his next goal—driving. We went out to a large retail parking lot and let him get behind the wheel and drive around for a while. We did this until he was comfortable, and one day he stayed in the driver's seat and drove us home. Tony is now driving on his own and only uses a single cane rather than the quad cane! He continues to set goals for himself and works hard to achieve 10,000 or more steps each day.

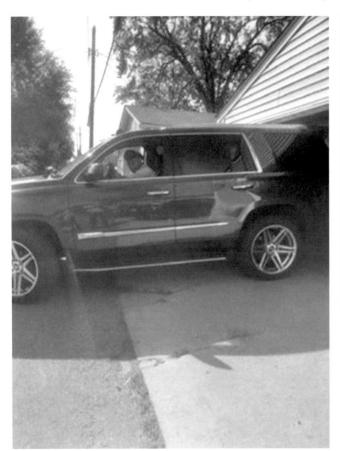
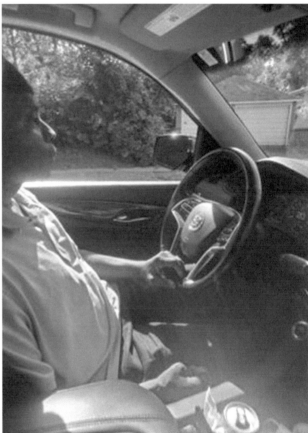

Glory to God and thanks to the prayers of the saints and help of all the wonderful caretakers, Tony's condition is improving every day. He is stronger, active, independent, and in high spirits.

To the readers of this book, it is my sincere hope and prayer that this testimony provides you with a fundamental understanding and education, as well as inspiration, and encouragement to live a healthier lifestyle and to endure and overcome any difficulty you may face.

References

Written by American Heart Association editorial staff and reviewed by science and medicine advisors. "African Americans and Heart Disease." American Heart Association. 31 July 2015,

https://www.heart.org/en/health-topics/consumer-healthcare/what-is-cardiovascular-disease/african-americans-and-heart-disease-stroke

American Stroke Association. https://www.stroke.org/en/about-stroke/types-of-stroke

National Institute of Neurological Disorders and Stroke (NINDS). "Brain Basics: Preventing Stroke." NIH Publication No. 11-3440b, 16 April 2020,

https://www.ninds.nih.gov/Disorders/Patient-Caregiver-Education/Preventing-Stroke

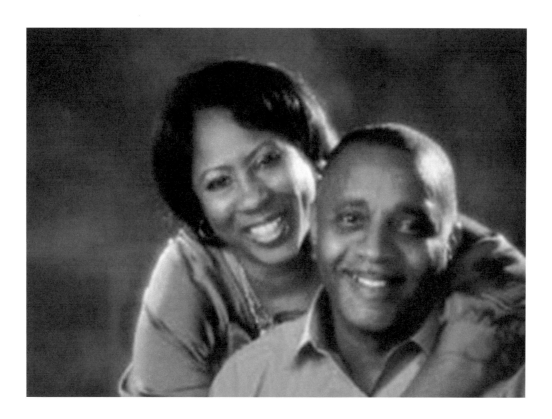

Anthony (Tony) Williams & Connie Thomas Williams

Tony & Connie Williams are ordained pastors and serve at Lighthouse Outreach Ministries in Saint Paul, Minnesota. They have been married for 27 years and blessed with five adult children and five grandchildren. In addition to being husband and wife, they are best friends and business partners, having owned and operated two fast food franchises for 15 years and worked in the food service industry for over 30 years.

God has blessed and anointed them to live the Word, walk in the Word and share the Word by demonstrations of faith principles.

Printed in the United States
by Baker & Taylor Publisher Services